Yaneisy Domínguez González
Amanda Pozas Ravelo
Katia Trujillo Castellanos

Cystic Fibrosis

Yaneisy Domínguez González
Amanda Pozas Ravelo
Katia Trujillo Castellanos

Cystic Fibrosis

Psychological and social characteristics in pediatric patients.

ScienciaScripts

SUMMARY:

Cystic Fibrosis (CF) is a genetic disease with a high degree of severity and progression that generates emotional damage in patients and family members. In order to characterize from a psycho-social point of view the patients with a diagnosis of Cystic Fibrosis treated at the "José Luis Miranda" Pediatric Hospital in 2021, a descriptive observational study was carried out, with a cross-sectional, quantitative and qualitative approach. The universe and the sample consisted of 14 patients. Instruments were applied to measure anxiety, depression, self-esteem, disease status and search for areas of conflict, interests, motivations, aspirations, needs, family ties, school activity and interpersonal relationships. The patients were mainly of school age, especially adolescents, with a slight female predominance, characteristics that were not significantly associated with affective symptoms. The mean values of anxiety as a trait and between medium and high as a state were frequent, with a predominance of patients without depression or with mild depression, with a slightly higher frequency in the female sex. In dysfunctional families, there was evidence of high levels of anxiety as a state, and no relationship was found between affective symptoms and the severity of the disease or self-esteem. The qualitative analysis identified that dysfunctional families, with difficulties in coping with the disease, generated higher levels of anxiety in the patient and difficulties with self-esteem, although not with the evolution of the disease.

Index

INTRODUCTION: 3

OBJECTIVE: 7

THEORETICAL FRAMEWORK: 8

METHODOLOGICAL DESIGN: 18

DISCUSSION OF RESULTS: 38

CONCLUSIONS: 45

RECOMMENDATIONS: 46

BIBLIOGRAPHICAL REFERENCES: 47

ANNEX 59

INTRODUCTION:

Cystic Fibrosis (CF) is a genetic disease in which the evolution of medicine over the last decades is reflected. Since 1936, when Fanconi published the description of a family with clinical features consisting of a "familial congenital fibromatosis of the pancreas with bronchiectasis" in a European medical journal. Also, almost at the same time on the other side of the Atlantic, a similar study was published by Andersen in 1938, describing "cystic fibrosis of the pancreas and its relations to celiac disease". CF has gone from being an exclusively infantile disease to being an adult disease as well.

Faber, in 1944, was the first to state that this disease was generalized and affected the mucus-secreting glands and suggested the name "mucoviscidosis".[1,2]

Di Sant'Agnese, Darling, Perera and Ethel Shea, published in 1953 the results of a study, carried out on the basis that in cystic fibrosis of the pancreas there could be a pluriglandular disorder including the sweat glands, thus being the first to describe the abnormal electrolyte composition of sweat in CF.

In 1959 Gibson and Cooke described a method for the determination of electrolyte concentration by means of the pilocarpine iontophoresis sweat stimulation test, which allowed confirming clinical suspicions of the disease.[3]

Later in 1963, Shwachman described a practical and simple method using the measurement of sweat conductivity, this method allowed the possibility of performing a sweat test of less complication and extend its practice massively.[4]

These and other research efforts culminated in the localization of the gene responsible for CF by a group of researchers led by Lap-Chee, Tsui and John R Riordan, *Hospital for Sick Children*, Toronto, and Francis S. Collins, University of Michigan in 1989.[5]

Cystic fibrosis (CF) is a genetic disease with autosomal recessive inheritance, i.e. an individual must have loss-of-function mutations in both copies of his or her CFTR (*cystic fibrosis transmembrane conductance regulator*) gene to manifest the disease. [6,7]

The incidence of the disease is about 1:3,300 live newborns in populations defined as Caucasian and the frequency of healthy carriers of a mutation (not identifiable by clinical symptoms or sweat test elevations) is 1:25.[3,4,8]

In the United States, Europe, and Australia the incidence is 1 in 3000 to 5000 children. [9,10] It is more common in Hispanic countries with a significant number (1 in 7000), Africa and America (1 in 12,000), and other American nations. [4,5,11,] This disease rarely occurs in individuals of Asian origin. Worldwide there are an estimated 100,000 affected individuals.[12] In Mexico an average of 400 to 600 new cases are reported annually.[6]

No epidemiological studies have been carried out in Spain, so an incidence of 1/2500 is assumed.[13] and Cuba report CF incidence of (1/3,862).[14]

It is a multi-organ disease and the symptoms result from deficient chloride transport across exocrine gland epithelia due to the absence or dysfunction of the CFTR 130 chloride channel. [1,2, 4,7]

It is characterized by a wide range in its clinical expression and a great variation in the severity and degree of progression of the different organs involved. In its classic and most common form it manifests as chronic obstructive pulmonary disease and exocrine pancreatic insufficiency (PI). In its non-classical form it manifests as chronic obstructive pulmonary disease, pancreatic insufficiency, malnutrition, elevated sweat chloride and infertility in males due to obstructive azoospermia. A significant number of patients are mildly affected and diagnosis is relatively common in older children, adolescents and even adults.[10,11,13]

Lung damage in these patients occurs progressively from birth, so the prognosis of these patients depends largely on early diagnosis and adequate respiratory and nutritional management. [7,10,15-17]

Cystic Fibrosis presents great variability in its severity and has gone from being a pediatric and fatal disease to become chronic and multisystemic with a median expected survival of almost 40 years at present. [4,8]

Due to improved survival, in the last 20 years the measurement of health-related quality of life (HRQoL), defined as a multidimensional construct that includes various patient-reported factors (physical, psychological and social functioning, symptoms, treatment burden and body image, among others), has gained importance. Its measurement provides information about the impact of treatment on the subject's symptoms and daily dynamics, allows measuring and comparing outcomes after the application of certain treatments and helps to better understand the differences in daily activities of patients with a similar degree of severity of the disease that cannot be obtained through somatic tests.[8]

This is associated with the way in which the patient copes with the disease and its treatment. The type of depressive coping has been related to the lack of therapeutic compliance, the development of anxiety and depression and the adoption of risk behaviors, with increased morbidity and decreased survival.[9]

Different authors have observed that anxious and depressive symptoms are elevated in patients with CF compared to the general population, and the presence of depressive symptoms has been associated with a worse respiratory functional status and HRQoL.[18-21]

The life of a patient with CF is marked from the time of diagnosis by the need to undergo constant medical check-ups, follow a demanding and demanding treatment and, in spite of this, be alert to the signs of the degenerative process of the disease, which generates a high degree of stress that has consequences at the psychological level. This can provoke emotions of helplessness, handicap, anguish, low self-esteem, anger and rage which, in turn, can lead to the appearance of emotional blockage, depression, anxiety and isolation.[23-26]

At the "José Luis Miranda" Provincial Pediatric Hospital, 22 patients with fibrocystic fibrosis are currently being treated, including infants and adults. Before the creation of shock therapies for the treatment of CF, most of the patients died before they reached 14 years of age. Survival has been increasing in the last two decades after the introduction in the country of new therapeutic protocols that include medications and more advanced respiratory physiotherapy techniques.

The interdisciplinary team that takes care of patients with Cystic Fibrosis in the Villa Clara nucleus is formed by highly qualified personnel, especially in the clinical area, nevertheless and in spite of the attention that they have received from the psychological point of view, it is perceived that the actions that have been carried out in this important area are still not enough. This situation becomes more complex because each patient and family behaves differently, and the social environment is also different.

Since no research has been conducted to characterize patients with Cystic Fibrosis from the psycho-social point of view, and taking into account the importance of addressing these aspects due to their impact on the evolution and prognosis, the present study was conducted to answer the following scientific problem:

What are the psychological and social characteristics of patients with Cystic Fibrosis treated at the "José Luis Miranda" Pediatric Hospital from July to December 2021?

OBJECTIVE:

To characterize from the psycho-social point of view the patients with a diagnosis of Cystic Fibrosis treated at the Pediatric Hospital "José Luis Miranda".

THEORETICAL FRAMEWORK:

Cystic fibrosis (CF) is a chronic, progressive, genetic disease that affects various organs, such as the exocrine cells of the respiratory tract, pancreas, liver, sweat ducts and reproductive system. The pulmonary pathophysiology is characterized by a deficiency or defect in the function of the transmembrane conductance regulator protein (CFTR). This causes an abnormality in the regulation of periciliary fluid volume, with decreased mucociliary clearance and the consequent production of plugs and pulmonary obstruction.[10, 11, 13,15]

Productive cough is a universal symptom in CF, which becomes chronic as the disease progresses. Respiratory exacerbations are associated with increased cough and expectoration, loss of appetite and impaired exercise capacity, resulting in school absenteeism. Exacerbations become more frequent as the disease progresses and cough becomes a regular symptom. [7,27-29]

Furthermore, cough has a direct influence on survival and is an important measure of disease progression and treatment efficacy. Clinical experience suggests that chronic cough interferes with the physical, emotional and social dimensions of the patient. Consequently, the patient's quality of life worsens considerably and his or her social relationships are affected.[30]

The disease is characterized by thickening of the mucus produced by the exocrine glands inducing sino-pulmonary involvement with progressive pulmonary damage, pancreatic insufficiency and therefore malabsorption syndrome, with consequent malnutrition, male sterility due to atrophy of the vas deferens and elevation of electrolytes in the sweat. Depending on the mutations involved there is a great diversity of clinical forms. [15,17,29]

Studies in families with CF began in 1985 using genetic markers that were located in the CFTR gene region. This was a breakthrough for families as it was possible to approach carrier detection from the nuclear family. The CFTR (cystic fibrosis transmembrane conductance regulator) gene was identified in 1989 in the 7q31 region of chromosome 7. The most frequent mutation is due to the loss of the amino acid phenylalanine at codon 508 (F508del). By immunohistochemical techniques, CFTR messenger RNA has been identified in sweat glands, pancreas, intestinal crypts, bile ducts and, in large quantities, in renal tubules, where the disease is not expressed, perhaps due to the existence of an alternative chloride channel. Since then, more than 1600 mutations have been identified, permanently updated in the Cystic Fibrosis Genetic Analysis Consortium (CFGAC) database.[5-7,31,32]

Three basic options are currently involved in the diagnostic confirmation of CF: prenatal and neonatal diagnosis, sweat test and genetic study.[1] Tests for neonatal screening for CF are based on the presence of elevated concentrations of cationic immunoreactive trypsin (IRT) in serum, an enzyme produced in the pancreas. [33,34] According to the European Consensus, a diagnosis of "classical cystic fibrosis" is established in the presence of at least one phenotypic feature of CF, together with a sweat chloride concentration > 60 mmol/l. In these patients, two disease-causing mutations in the CFTR gene are usually detected, they may or may not have pancreatic insficiency, and their clinical course is variable. A diagnosis of "non-classical or atypical cystic fibrosis" is established if at least one of the phenotypic features and a borderline sweat test result (chlorine 30-60 mmol/l) is find along with the detection of two mutations and/or an altered nasal potential difference (NPD).[15]

The pneumological follow-up of the patient with cystic fibrosis should be supported by the following points:

1. Clinical. At each visit, the patient will be examined and the presence of respiratory symptoms will be recorded.[15]

2. Imaging tests. Chest X-ray may be normal, but it is advisable to perform it as soon as the patient is diagnosed. [17]

High-resolution computed tomography (HRCT), more accurately identifies areas of focal involvement and is able to detect bronchiectasis in smaller bronchial ramifications.[7]

3. Microbiology. Microbiological surveillance by sputum culture will be performed every 1-2 months and in respiratory exacerbations.

4. Pulmonary function and blood gases. It is convenient to perform FEF, FEV (expired volume in the first second) and a bronchodilator test, to include it or not in the treatment according to the response obtained.[35]

Maintenance therapy aims to prevent chronic Pseudomona aeruginosa infection or colonization, reduce the number and severity of pulmonary exacerbations and slow the infectious-inflammatory cycle that leads to irreversible lung damage. [1,2]

Cystic fibrosis disease and death are primarily due to progressive destruction of the lung disease resulting in respiratory failure.[4]

Currently, prevention is not possible once the baby is born. In babies with two abnormal CF genes, the disease is already present at birth. Couples who have one or more children with CF in their families can be tested to determine if they are carriers of the disease; if they are, they should ideally be counseled by physicians and specialists in order to make decisions about the likelihood of having another child with CF. [5,33]

Since the first publications on CF patients, at which time less than 50% of patients lived more than one year, survival has clearly improved. According to data from the American Cystic Fibrosis Foundation patient registry, median survival was 4 years in the 1960s, reaching 27 in 1985 and 35.9 years in 2009.[12]

The life expectancy rate has evolved similarly for much of Europe, with the exception of the least developed countries, where significantly lower figures are reported, since this mortality indicator tends to vary mainly according to the extent and quality of care provided by the health systems.[13]

Thanks to these data, it can be affirmed that CF is the disease in which the prognosis of patients and their quality of life have changed most notably in the last three decades. As a consequence of this improvement in the life expectancy of the disease, various comorbidities are emerging, among which depression and anxiety stand out. [18,21,22]

Several studies,[36-39] have shown that patients with chronic diseases have a higher risk of depression and anxiety. CF is no exception as a chronic disease and also presents higher levels of depression and anxiety in both patients and parent caregivers. [40,41]

Studies in the general population indicate that both depression and anxiety are associated with a worse clinical course. It has been shown that these higher rates of depression and anxiety can have both direct and indirect negative consequences on the clinical course of the underlying disease. [39,42]

It is known that depressed patients are less adherent to correct treatment guidelines, are more likely to miss check-ups, report poorer scores in different areas of quality of life in specifically designed questionnaires, use more health care resources or incur greater health care costs, and are also more likely to develop risky behaviors. [41,43]

To date, studies on the impact of depression and anxiety in CF patients have been limited by small sample sizes, samples that could provide biased estimates of symptom rates, and that have used measures that confounded symptoms of depression with those of chronic illness.[29,36]

Psychological and social aspects:

CF is a disease where the family is the main responsible for the children's compliance with the treatment. If they do everything right, they survive longer. The disease can affect several areas of their lives, both at a personal, family and social level.[44]

Those affected by Q.F. constitute a group of mostly children and adolescents, whose existence takes place in a significant way in the spheres of the education system, from where they try to acquire an essential component for the development of the human being such as education.

However, the progressive evolution of the disease may hinder an adequate development of education. Likewise, unexpected relapses, together with frequent medical check-ups, may generate involuntary school absenteeism in these students in a variable degree of incidence depending on the case.

This forced absence from the classroom makes it difficult for the F.Q. sufferer to follow the curricular program with due regularity, which has a negative impact on his or her school performance or even prevents him or her from attending evaluative tests.[45]

One of the most important indicators of social integration is labor integration. For people with CF, this is a new field in their lives, since until not long ago the average person with CF did not reach working age. The situation of people entering employment for the first time who are affected by CF brings with it a series of difficulties that must be equated with those of young people who do not have CF. There are limitations in accessing certain jobs because the disease itself hinders their performance and will even have an impact on the deterioration of their health.

They should not be in work environments with fumes or where substances such as dust from any material or chemicals are released, since this type of environment harms the pulmonary condition they already suffer from. It is not advisable to work full day or night shifts, since they can make it difficult to follow the daily treatment. It is advisable to have a flexible schedule, since there will be frequent absences from work due to check-ups, treatments and/or relapses. Due to the treatment and the antibiotic medication they take, they get tired earlier than other people, and they have a limited pulmonary capacity, so it will be very difficult for them to perform heavy physical work.
9,21

Interpersonal Relationships:

Family experience of the disease:

The expectations that parents have placed on the desired child are shattered by the unexpected diagnosis of a chronic and degenerative disease such as Cystic Fibrosis, the emotions that usually appear at this time are usually: worry, anguish, guilt, sadness, fear, frustration. [20,21]

If the adaptation to the new situation is carried out with appropriate strategies and the disease is accepted, the family structure need not be affected, but if this does not occur, there is a risk of conflict, tension and instability.

The difficult role of the parents at this stage will be mediated by the readjustment of their lives to new habits in terms of diet, breathing exercises, taking medication. This readjustment involves, in some cases, losses: some mothers may stop working, their partners may reduce or even stop going out with friends, they may stop doing pleasurable activities, thus aggravating negative and unpleasant emotions due to the lack of moments of satisfaction, and in other cases the parents were already separated. [45,47]

Relationships outside the family nucleus

There is a high degree of concealment of information about the patient's disease and daily activities (such as physiotherapy) from study and/or work colleagues, creating not only barriers in communication and hindering the relationship, but also, in some cases, as can happen at work, suffering adverse environmental circumstances (for example, not saying anything when colleagues smoke too much). [48]

The feeling of being different and the complication of explaining such a "rare" disease and the characteristics of its treatment, make the patient not to talk about it with his peers or simply say that he has asthma or "stomach problems". This means that, on many occasions, they do not participate in the same activities due to embarrassment about the treatment (having to do physiotherapy, application of aerosols or, to a lesser extent, taking medication) or due to the characteristics of the disease (morning coughs, when going to the bathroom), which creates a certain social isolation that is important to treat. [49]

Relationships with the partner:

CF is no longer a pediatric disease, so as the adolescent grows older, he or she encounters new needs and problems, such as the decision to form a couple. In most cases, the most serious pairing takes place at an older age. The choice of a partner is sometimes made within the group of friends, due to the already existing trust.

Once the sentimental bond is formed, there are often mixed feelings: wanting to share everything with the other person, but not knowing how to express their feelings about the disease or the future, and even not feeling understood. At first, fear of intimacy and embarrassment about how the peculiarities of the disease or the treatment may influence the other person. Anxiety about being able or not, and/or wanting or not, to start a family. All these normal feelings that you are now facing must be dealt with and understood, so that they can be properly managed and do not become an obstacle in the couple's relationship. Therefore, it is necessary the collaboration of professionals to help create guidelines for communication, management of feelings, expression of them. [40,43,44, 49,50]

Depressive symptoms have been assessed primarily in observational studies of different CF patient populations. Researchers have used the Beck Youth Inventory to assess depression, anxiety, anger, problem behavior, and self-concept in children with CF.[22] In addition, the Hospital Anxiety and Depression Scale (HADS),[36] the Mood and Feelings Questionnaire (MFQ), the Zung Self-Applied Depression Scale (SDS) and the Beck Depression Inventory[51] have been used in numerous clinical settings to assess the prevalence of depression in CF patients.[41,43,52,53]

Research suggests that people with CF, despite the burden of the disease and the treatments they carry, are psychologically well adjusted. Using questionnaires with physical and psychological dimensions, children and adults with CF generally scored lower than the healthy population on most physical dimensions, but had similar HRQoL on psychological dimensions[54,55] it is noteworthy that adolescents with CF were less likely than the general population to have a recognized mental disorder. [47,49]

This seems contrary to the expectation that people with life-threatening illnesses can have a good HRQoL. This could be due to a phenomenon known as "response switching". According to this phenomenon, a subject's lived reality always influences his or her expectations, and the mechanisms by which an individual evaluates or quantifies his or her HRQoL change in response to multiple factors. It would be a re-evaluation of the meaning of life and, therefore, an adaptation to changing conditions.[48]

Considering that mortality attributed to Cystic Fibrosis is high, due to the fact that it affects multiple organs and evolves in a chronic and progressive manner, is necessary to implement comprehensive and multidisciplinary care models that favor the follow-up and treatment of patients with the disease.

In addition, comprehensive care and a shared understanding of the pathology among professionals contribute to prolonging survival and reducing morbidity and mortality.

Multidisciplinary care is essential for the integration of knowledge, in order to impose permanent updating of scientific information, thus contributing to the development of intervention strategies, which improve survival and motivate the development of skills to cope with the treatment regimen.[7,47]

Since the diagnosis of cystic fibrosis, a psychological intervention is necessary to support the family with the impact that the chronic disease, its implications and expectations will have on the child and his caregivers. Since CF survival estimates are steadily increasing, long-term treatment in this area is of great interest in order to cope better with this disease. Psychological interventions should target emotional and social adaptations, treatment compliance, and quality of life. Often people with CF and other family members need help in psychological and emotional adjustment, mainly in aspects of coping with the disease or genetic risk, improving dietary intake, and improving the effectiveness of respiratory physiotherapy. Key moments are diagnosis, adolescence, sexuality linked to fertility, awareness of early mortality and terminal stage.[54-56]

From childhood, these interventions should be focused on the characteristics of the stage of the life cycle, since according to the age different psychological manifestations are produced that will have to be addressed, from childhood to adulthood, according to the evolutionary crises that are experienced at each stage, which in the case of these people will be influenced by the perception of health-illness, signs and symptoms that are being experienced, treatment and implications for day-to-day activities.[40]

There are reports of specific educational or behavioral psychological interventions aimed at specific treatment concerns during the chronic phase. [45,57] There is some evidence that behavioral interventions can improve emotional outcomes in CF patients and caregivers. Although there are no studies that demonstrate a statistically significant association between psychological interventions and clinical improvements,[41,58] it is necessary to address psychological aspects in the treatment to ensure the success of the clinical intervention and a comprehensive approach that not only focuses on the disease but also on the person and his/her family.

The social integration of patients with chronic disease represents a great challenge in our society, technological advances in medicine have allowed an early clinical diagnosis and greater life expectancy in patients with chronic pathology such as Cystic Fibrosis. This disease that is diagnosed in childhood should be approached by health professionals and community considering the integration in daily life activities, for this is relevant the acceptance of prevention measures that the patient and environment acquire associated to the individual manifestations that are producing the disease and/or treatment, in order to maintain a life as normal as possible within their capabilities that allows them to have fun, attend school, higher education or work activity depending on the stage of life cycle they are living. Another aspect in the social area to consider are the social aids that the community will give to patients and family. [58-60]

METHODOLOGICAL DESIGN:

A descriptive observational, cross-sectional, cross-sectional study was conducted with a quantitative and qualitative approach in patients with a diagnosis of Cystic Fibrosis treated in Villa Clara during the second semester of the year 2021.

The study population consisted of 14 patients with a diagnosis of Cystic Fibrosis who were attended by the multidisciplinary team of the "José Luis Miranda" Pediatric Hospital, with an equal number of patients in the sample and who met the following inclusion criteria.

Inclusion criteria:

-        Patients older than 9 years of age to whom it was possible to apply the established evaluation instruments.

-        Patients whose family members were willing to participate with prior informed consent in the case of minors, or who wished to participate in the case of adults (Annex 1. Informed Consent Form).

Exclusion criteria:

•   Death during the study.

•   Study abandonment

All patients were administered several established and validated instruments to evaluate psychological and social aspects in two consecutive consultations (October and December) in the year 2021. In addition, medical records were reviewed.

Data collection techniques:

•   Documentary review, a medical history review guide was prepared to extract age and sex.

•   To measure the level of anxiety, Ch.D. Spielberger's Trait-State Anxiety Inventory for Children was used. It was applied to patients older than 9 years old. Self-Assessment Inventory (Annex 2). The IDARE is a self-assessment inventory designed to assess two relatively independent forms of anxiety: anxiety as a state (transient emotional condition) and anxiety as a trait (relatively stable anxious propensity). Self-applied. Each has 20 items. In the IDARE-state, there are 10 positive anxiety items (i.e., the higher the score, the higher the anxiety) and 10 negative items. In the trait scale there are 13 positive and 7 negative items. The response form ranges from 0 to 4 in both subscales. In the State Scale the subject is instructed to answer how he/she feels at the present moment in relation to the formulated items, and how he/she generally feels in relation to the items of the Trait Anxiety Scale.

Correction and Interpretation

For scoring, the score achieved in each item was calculated. The key was used, so as to know which groups of annotations are added, since some propositions are formulated in a direct way, as evaluating anxiety (e.g. I am nervous) and others in an inverse way (e.g. I am calm). A formula was then used, whose final result allowed the subject to be placed in different levels of anxiety for each scale, being Low, Moderate or High.

It provided a state anxiety score and a trait anxiety score, which take values from 20 to 80 points.

IDARE qualification strategy

A. State 3+4+6+7+9+12+13+14+14+17+18= A

1+2+5+8+10+11+15+16+19+20= B

(A-B)+50=

_______High (> = 45)

_______Medium (30-44)

_______Low (< = 30)

A. Trait 22+23+24+25+28+28+29+29+31+32+32+34+35+35+37+37+38+40

=A 21+26+27+30+33+35+39 =B.

(A-B)+35=

_______High (> = 45)

Medium (30-44)

Low (< = 30)

- The Zung and Conde test was used to measure the level of depression (Appendix 3). It was applied to patients between the ages of 9 years to adulthood. The Zung Depression Self-Scale dates from 1965; the version used corresponds to the adaptation made by Zung and Conde, 1969; it is a 20-item questionnaire, which investigates the frequency of occurrence in a subject of sadness, hopelessness, crying, self-punishment, dissatisfaction, suicidal rumination, irritability, indecision, sleep, physical fatigue, weight loss, loss of appetite, constipation, tachycardia, sex, diurnal variation, slowing down.

Scoring Table. Zung-Conde Depression Test:

Diagnosis	Annotation
No Depression	20-33
Mild depression	34-40
Moderate depression 41-54	41-47 Medium neurotic depression
	48-54 High neurotic depression
Severe depression	55-80

- The FF-SIL test (Pérez, De la Cuesta, Louro and Bayarre) was used to measure the perception of family functioning (Annex 4). It was applied to all patients. Validated in Cuba since 1994, it offers an easy application and qualification for the care team, providing high reliability and validity, which indicates that the test aims to measure through the following dimensions:

1. **Cohesion**: Physical and emotional family union when facing different situations, and in the decision making process of daily tasks.

2. **Harmony:** Correspondence between individual interests and needs, with those of the family in a positive emotional balance.

3.   **Communication:** Members are able to convey their experiences, and knowledge clearly and directly.

4.   **Adaptability:** Ability to change power structure, role relationships and rules in a situation that requires it.

5.   **Affectivity:** Ability of members to experience and demonstrate positive feelings and emotions to each other.

6.   **Role:** Each family member fulfills the responsibilities and functions negotiated by the family nucleus.

7.   **Permeability:** Ability to offer and receive experiences from other families and institutions.

The final score is obtained from the sum of the points for each item. Scores will be awarded according to the following scale:

Almost never - 1 point.
Rarely - 2 points. Sometimes- 3 points.

Often - 4 points. Almost always- 5 points.

This test allows the family to be classified into 4 types:

1.   Functional family- 70-57 points.

2.   Moderately functional family-56-43 points.

3.   Dysfunctional family-42-28 points.

4.   Severely dysfunctional family- 27-14 points (6)

•   A clinical history review guide was prepared to extract the necessary data for the application of the Shwachman Score (Annex 5). It was applied to all patients.

•   To measure the level of self-esteem (Self-esteem questionnaire, Annex 6). It was applied to all patients. This questionnaire was made in 1996, at the Psychology Department of the Central University of Las Villas (UCLV), and it has 25 simple sentences that reflect aspects related to self-acceptance and self-esteem of adolescents. It is adjusted to the characteristics of Cuban adolescents. For the scoring, the number of sentences that do not correspond to the normal or adequate response was determined and is taken to the following scale:

From 0 to 5: very high self-esteem.

From 6 to 11: high self-esteem.

From 12 to 20 low self-esteem.

Above 20: very low self-esteem.

In addition, qualitative interpretation of the results was performed.

• To search for areas of conflict, interests, motivations, aspirations, needs, family ties, school activity and interpersonal relationships, the Sentence Completion Test (ROTTER) was used (Appendix 7). It was applied to patients aged between 13 years and adulthood.

Description of the test: It consists of presenting the subject with the beginning of 56 sentences dealing with multiple aspects, allowing him/her to complete them spontaneously.

Objectives: To explore the subject's areas of conflict, aspirations, motivations, interests, needs, family ties, school activity and interpersonal relationships.

Materials: Sheet of paper with 48 incomplete ideas.

Procedure: Try to complete the sentences to express your ideas, write the first idea that comes to your mind, don't think too much. There are no right or wrong answers.

Scoring: The analysis of this technique was based on the suggestions made by Fernando Glez Rey (1982) by virtue of a qualitative assessment that directs the analysis of each of the items and their scoring. Instead, units of information of a relevant nature were established from whose interpretation the integral results of the diagnosis are obtained, considering for this purpose the frequency of appearance of the revealed contents.

For the analysis, areas or spheres were created (family, personal, school, social) and interests were classified as fears related to the disease.

Of the 48 items:

8 are directed to the sexual sphere. 4 to the school sphere.

4 to the family sphere

26 are directed to the personal and relational sphere.
6 are mattress questions.

In the same sphere, one sentence refers to the aspired and the other to the achieved. The prevalence criterion in each sphere is touched upon. Patient assessments of their personality, aspirations, goals and how they experience their symptoms can be explored.

The labor sphere is not evaluated because it is not adapted to the age of the sample and the objectives of the research.

• To look for areas of conflict, the Juvenile Problems Inventory was applied (Annex 8). It was applied to patients over 13 years of age. These instruments have a standardized process for their application, and their results, both those resulting from a quantitative method of qualification, as well as those derived from the qualitative analysis of the professional, have to be contrasted with the observation and general information obtained from the subject; that is to say that the evaluation instruments are always working tools, and even more so in children and adolescents, because they are people in full development of their possibilities and are more exposed in their development, than adults, to various contexts that determine it as the school and social, in addition to the family environment.

Triangulation of information: This was a qualitative analysis technique to be used from the data collected in the observation, survey, interview and documentary review, when contrasted with the results obtained from the quantitative point of view.

Mathematical-Statistical

Percentage analysis and descriptive statistics: In the evaluation and quantitative and qualitative processing of the data obtained in the results of each stage of the research.

All this was carried out taking into account the informed consent of all those involved in the study, for which an informed consent form was prepared and is attached (Annex 1).

Operationalization of the variables:

Variable	Scale	Description
Age	From 9 to 15 years old. Mayord e 15 years of age.	According to age at the time of the investigation.
Sex	Female Male	According to biological sex of belonging.
Trait anxiety	Low Medium High	The patient reflects relatively stable anxious propensity. Evaluated with the Trait-State Anxiety Inventory. for children IDARE, (Annex 2).

Anxiety state	Low Medium High	Unpleasant subjective experiential state involving expectation, anxiety, restlessness, apprehension, with no known causal basis or real object present, which may be accompanied by motor restlessness and neurovegetative disorders such as tachycardia, sweating, epigastric jumping, among others. There is an experiential, motor and behavioral expression. Evaluated with the Trait-State Anxiety Inventory for Children IDARE, (Annex 2).
Depression	No depression Mild Moderate Moderate Severe	State of unhappy dissatisfaction, characterized by sadness, given by a quantitative exaltation of affectivity towards the negative pole ranging from slight dejection to extreme sadness. Evaluated with Test of Zung and Conde (Annex 3).

Family functioning	Functional family Moderately functional family Dysfunctional family Severely dysfunctional family	The way in which the family system, as a group, is capable of facing crises, valuing the way in which expressions of affection are allowed, the individual growth of its members, and the interaction among them, based on respect, autonomy and the space of the other. Evaluated with the Family Functioning questionnaire (Annex 4).
Statusof of the disease	Excellent Good Good Mild Moderate Moderate Severe	Evaluated with theGuide at Medical History According to the results of the score. Shwachman (Annex 5).
Self-esteem	High Medium Under	Statusof self-acceptance and self-esteem of adolescents , evaluated with questionnaire
		self-esteem, (Annex 6).
Are as of human behavior	Personal Area Family Area Social Area School Area Sexual Area	Evaluated with the Rotter Adolescent Sentence Completion Test questionnaire (Appendix 7) and the Juvenile Problems Inventory (JPI) (Appendix 8).

RESULTS:

A total of 14 pediatric patients with Cystic Fibrosis are included in the research, their distribution according to the presence of anxiety as a trait and state in relation to age can be observed in Table 1.

Table 1. Patients with Cystic Fibrosis according to age and anxiety as a trait and state. José Luis Miranda Pediatric Hospital. 2021

Age **Anxiety**		9 to 15 years		Greater than 15 years		Total	
		N°	%	N°	%	N°	%
Trait anxiety	Under	1	7,14	1	7,14	2	14,29
	Medium	6	42,86	4	28,57	10	71,43
	High	0	0,00	2	14,29	2	14,29
Anxiety state	Under	1	7,14	1	7,14	2	14,29
	Medium	3	21,43	3	21,43	6	42,86
	High	3	21,43	3	21,43	6	42,86

Source: Medical records.

	X^2	
Trait anxiety and age	2,4000	p = 0,3012
Anxiety status and age	0,0000	p = 1,0000

At the time of the investigation 7 patients were aged between 9 and 15 years and 7 were older than 15 years, which represented 50 % in each group.

Anxiety as a trait had a medium level of intensity in 71.43 % and was predominant in all ages, with 42.86 % in patients aged 9 to 15 years and 28.57 % in those older than 15 years, so that no dependence between the degree of anxiety as a trait and age is corroborated, p = 0.3012.

Anxiety as a state was manifested with a high level in 6 patients and similarly 6 presented a medium level, in both cases constituting 42.86 %, only 2 patients presented a low level for 14.29 %. The distribution of anxiety as a state was equal in the age groups, p = 1.000.

Table 2 shows the distribution of patients with Cystic Fibrosis with respect to age and the presence of depression. Six cases did not present depression, which represented 42.86 %, 4 of them without depression were between 9 and 15 years old for 28.57 % and 2 were older than 15 years old for 14.29 %.

Cystic Fibrosis patients according to age and depression.
José Luis Miranda Pediatric Hospital. 2021

| Depression | Age | | | | | |
| | 9 to 15 years | | Greater than 15 years | | Total | |
	N°	%	N°	%	N°	%
No depression	4	28,57	2	14,29	6	42,86
Slight	2	14,29	3	21,43	5	35,71
Moderate	1	7,14	1	7,14	2	14,29
Severa	0	0,00	1	7,14	1	7,14
Total	7	50,00	7	50,00	14	100

Source: Medical records.

$X^2 = 1.8667$ p = 0,6505

Mild depression was manifested in 5 patients who constituted 35.71 %, of these 2 with age between 9 and 15 years (14.29 %) and 3 older than 15 (21.43 %).

Moderate depression was evidenced in 2 patients (14.29 %) with equal distribution according to age and severe depression was manifested in 1 patient older than 15 years constituting 7.14 %.

There was no dependence between depression and age in pediatric patients with Cystic Fibrosis, p = 0.6505.

Cystic Fibrosis patients according to sex and psychopathies.
José Luis Miranda Pediatric Hospital. 2021.

Affective Symptoms		Sex				Total	
		Male		Female			
		N°	%	N°	%	N°	%
Trait anxiety	Under	0	0,00	2	14,29	2	14,29
	Medium	4	28,57	6	42,86	10	71,43
	High	2	14,29	0	0,00	2	14,29
Anxiety state	Under	0	0,00	2	14,29	2	14,29
	Medium	2	14,29	4	28,57	6	42,86
	High	4	28,57	2	14,29	6	42,86
Depression	No depression	4	28,57	2	14,29	6	42,86
	Slight	1	7,14	4	28,57	5	35,71
	Moderate	1	7,14	1	7,14	2	14,29
	Severa	0	0,00	1	7,14	1	7,14

Source: Medical records.

Trait anxiety and gender	$X^2 = 4.2000$	$p = 0,1225$
Anxiety status and gender	$X^2 = 3.1111$	$p = 0,2111$
Depression and sex	$X^2 = 3.2472$	$p = 0,3551$

The distribution of affective symptoms in relation to sex is shown in the table below.

3. Anxiety as a trait predominated with medium intensity values in both males (28.57 %) and females (42.86 %). Although in males 2 cases (14.29 %) presented a high level and on the contrary in females 2 cases (14.29 %) presented a low level. Trait anxiety had a similar distribution in both sexes, p = 0.1225.

In the male sex, anxiety as a state with high level was present in 4 patients that constituted 28.57 %, however in the female sex anxiety as a state with medium intensity predominated in 4 cases (28.57 %), however the distribution of anxiety as a state did not depend significantly on sex, p = 0.2111.

As for depression, depression was not evident in 4 male patients (28.57 %), mild in 1 case (7.14 %) and moderate in 1 patient (7.14 %). In the females, mild depression was observed in 4 of these for 28.57 %, in 2 cases it was not evidenced (14.29 %) and it was moderate in 1 patient (7.14 %) and severe in 1 case (7.14 %).

Table 4 relates depression and anxiety as a trait and state to family functioning.

Of the total of 14 patients with cystic fibrosis, 8 (57.14 %) had moderately functional family functioning, of these, 5 cases had a medium level of anxiety as a trait for 35.71 %, in 2 patients low (14.29 %) and in 1 patient low (14.29 %) anxiety as a trait for 35.71 %.

%) and in 1 case high (7.14 %). Of the 6 patients with dysfunctional families, 5 presented anxiety as a trait with medium level for 35.71 %. Therefore, there was no significant association between trait anxiety and family functioning, p = 0.4169.

Patients with Cystic Fibrosis according to family functioning and affective symptoms. José Luis Miranda Pediatric Hospital. 2021

____
    Family functioning

Affective Symptoms		Moderately functional		Dysfunctional	
		N°	%	N°	%
Trait anxiety	Under	2	14,29	0	0,00
	Medium	5	35,71	5	35,71
	High	1	7,14	1	7,14
Anxiety state	Under	2	14,29	0	0,00
	Medium	5	35,71	1	7,14
	High	1	7,14	5	35,71
Depression	No depression	4	28,57	2	14,29
	Slight	3	21,43	2	14,29
	Moderate	0	0,00	2	14,29
	Severa	1	7,14	0	0,00

Source: Medical records.

Trait anxiety and family F	$X^2 = 1.7500$	$p = 0,4169$
Anxiety status and family F	$X^2 = 7.1944$	$p = 0,0274$
Depression and family F	$X^2 = 3.6556$	$p = 0,3011$

Anxiety as a state showed significant dependence, $p = 0.0274$, with family functioning. With moderately functional families and anxiety as a state with medium level we found 5 patients who constituted 35.71 %. However, of the 6 cases with dysfunctional families, 5 of them presented high levels of anxiety as a state, which made up 35.71% of the total.

Regarding depression, in children with moderately functional family, 4 patients did not present depression (28.57 %), in 3 cases it was mild (21.43 %) and in 1 patient it was severe (7.14 %).

In those who presented dysfunctional families, in 2 cases there was no depression, and similarly in 2 patients it was mild and in 2 patients moderate, all constituting

14.29 %. Depression did not show significant dependence with family functioning, p = 0.3011.

Table 5 shows the disease status and the presence of anxiety as a trait, state and depression.

In terms of disease status it was excellent in 2 patients (14.29 %), good in 5 cases (35.71 %), mild in 1 for 7.14 %, moderate in 4 which were 28.57 %, and severe in 2 patients (14.29 %).

Anxiety as a trait was not significantly associated (p = 0.9198) with disease severity, as the medium level of anxiety predominated in most patients regardless of the degree of the disease: 14.29 % with excellent evolution, 21.43 % classified as good, 7.14 % mild, 14.29 % moderate and 14.29 % severe.

Anxiety as a state was not significantly related to the severity of the disease, p = 0.9463. In general, it behaved in medium and high values.

Depression did not show dependence on the severity of the disease, p = 0.3011. It was absent in 3 cases considered in good status (21.43%) and 2 with moderate status (14.29%).

Patients with Cystic Fibrosis according to disease status and affective symptoms. José Luis Miranda Pediatric Hospital. 2021

Affective Symptoms		Disease status									
		Excellent		Good		Slight		Moderate		Serious	
		No.	%	No.	%	No.	%	No.	%	No.	%
Trait anxiety	Under	0	0,00	1	7,14	0	0,00	1	7,14	0	0,00
	Medium	2	14,29	3	21,43	1	7,14	2	14,29	2	14,29
	High	0	0,00	1	7,14	0	0,00	1	7,14	0	0,00
Anxiety state	Under	0	0,00	1	7,14	0	0,00	1	7,14	0	0,00
	Medium	1	7,14	2	14,29	1	7,14	1	7,14	1	7,14
	High	1	7,14	2	14,29	0	0,00	2	14,29	1	7,14
Depression	No depression	1	7,14	3	21,43	0	0,00	2	14,29	0	0,00

Slight	1	7,14	0	0,00	1	7,14	2	14,29	1	7,14
Moderate	0	0,00	1	7,14	0	0,00	0	0,00	1	7,14
Severa	0	0,00	1	7,14	0	0,00	0	0,00	0	0,00

Source: Medical records.

Trait anxiety and severity	$X^2 = 3.2200$	$p = 0,9198$
Anxiety status and severity	$X^2 = 2,8000$	$p = 0,9463$
Depression and severity	$X^2 = 3.6556$	$p = 0,3011$

Table 6 distributes the children with Cystic Fibrosis according to anxiety as a trait, state and depression in relation to self-esteem.

Six patients presented a high level of self-esteem (42.86 %), three patients a medium level (21.43 %), and three patients a low level of self-esteem (21.43 %).

%) and under 5 cases (35.71 %).

Anxiety as a trait was not significantly related to self-esteem, p =

0.256. Five patients (35.71 %) had high self-esteem and medium anxiety, 2 cases (14.29 %) had medium self-esteem and anxiety, and 3 cases (21.43 %) had low self-esteem and medium anxiety.

Anxiety as a state did not depend on the level of self-esteem, p = 0.113. Of the 6 patients with a high level of self-esteem, 4 (28.57 %) presented a high level of anxiety as a state and 2 medium levels (14.29 %). Of the 3 patients with medium level of self-esteem, 2, for 14.29 %, presented a high level of anxiety as a state. Of the 5 patients with a low level of self-esteem, 3 (21.43 %) presented a medium level of anxiety as a state and 2 a low level (14.29 %).

Patients with Cystic Fibrosis according to self-esteem and affective symptoms. José Luis Miranda Pediatric Hospital. 2021.

Affective Symptoms		Self-esteem					
		High		Medium		Under	
		N°	%	N°	%	N°	%
Trait anxiety	Under	0	0,00	0	0,00	2	14,29
	Medium	5	35,71	2	14,29	3	21,43
	High	1	7,14	1	7,14	0	0,00
Anxiety state	Under	0	0,00	0	0,00	2	14,29
	Medium	2	14,29	1	7,14	3	21,43
	High	4	28,57	2	14,29	0	0,00
Depression	No depression	3	21,43	1	7,14	2	14,29
	Slight	2	14,29	1	7,14	2	14,29
	Moderate	1	7,14	1	7,14	0	0,00
	Severa	0	0,00	0	0,00	1	7,14

Source: Medical records.

Trait anxiety and self-esteem $X^2 = 5.3200$ $p = 0,256$

Anxiety status and self-esteem $X^2 = 7.4667$ $p = 0,113$

Depression and self-esteem $X^2 = 3.4844$ $p = 0,746$

Depression did not show significant dependence on self-esteem, $p = 0.746$. Among the patients with high self-esteem, 3 (21.43%) did not present depression, in 2 cases it was mild (14.29%) and in 1 patient it was moderate (7.14%).

Cases with medium self-esteem level were distributed similarly with 1 patient each with no depression, mild depression and moderate depression, each representing 7.14 %.

Among patients with low self-esteem, 2 did not present depression (14.29%), 2 presented mild depression (14.29%) and 1 presented severe depression (7.14%).

Patients with Cystic Fibrosis according to affected areas of human behavior. José

Luis Miranda Pediatric Hospital. 2021.

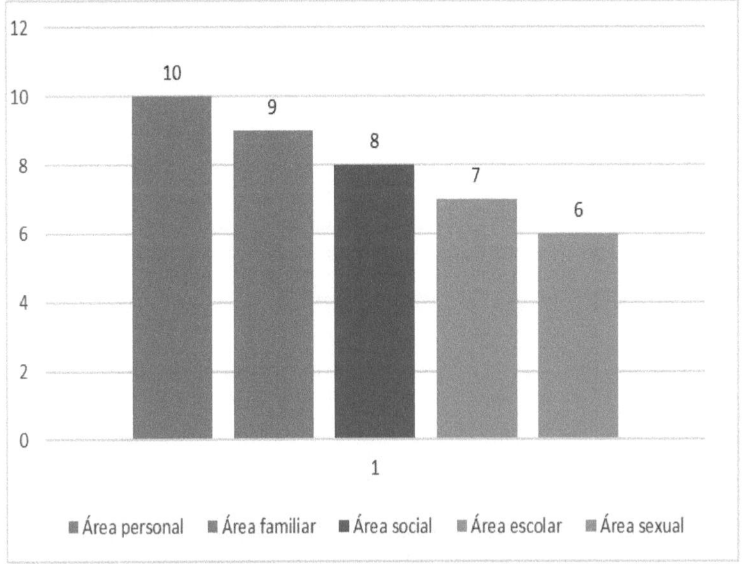

Graph 1 shows the distribution of children with Cystic Fibrosis according to the areas of human behavior affected. In order to determine them, the Rotter Infantile and the Juvenile Problems Inventory were applied, both from the age of 13 years, so the patients in this case were 10; all of them had affected the personal area, most of them had affected the family and social areas (9 and 8 patients respectively), in 7 there was evidenced affectation of the school area and in 6 of the sexual area.

Patients with Cystic Fibrosis according to the number of areas of human behavior affected. José Luis Miranda Pediatric Hospital. 2021.

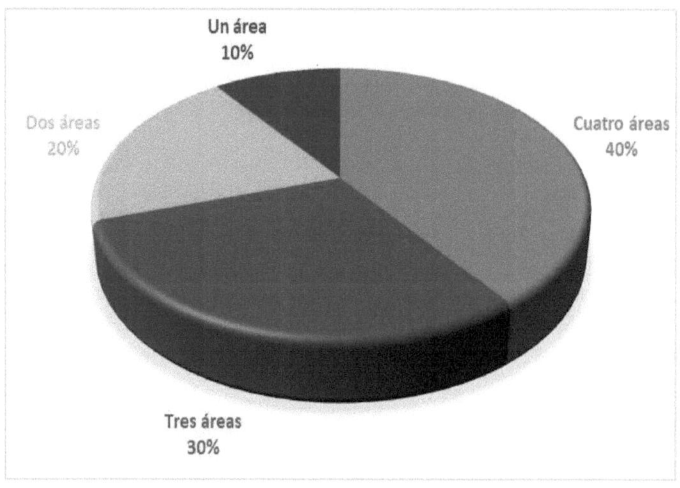

Of the total of 10 patients, 4 were affected in 4 areas of human behavior for 40%, 3 were affected in 3 areas of human behavior (30%), 2 (20%) in two areas of human behavior and 1 (10%) in one area of human behavior.

Integrative analysis of the psycho-affective and social situation of CF patients: In the family area, 6 dysfunctional families were found, generally due to crises related to separation of the parents, with abandonment of the work relationship, generally of the mothers, with social isolation. In these families there was evidence of a lack of psychological resources for coping with the disease and the treatment, presence of manifestations of overprotection and dependence that generate higher levels of depression and anxiety in the children. In some of these families, low family income and inadequate housing conditions were identified, factors that enhance the difficulties in the functioning of the family.

In the personal area, low self-esteem levels were identified in 5 patients, which corresponds to families classified as dysfunctional and 3 of these patients were adolescents, with a longer evolution of the disease. They manifest insecurity, uncertainty in relation to the future, fears and difficulties in social relations with peers and equals, in addition to dissatisfaction in the sexual sphere and poor physical development that generates dissatisfaction with their body image.

In the school area, low motivation for these activities was found mainly in patients with low self-esteem, although these difficulties were not identified in most of them, observing adequate school performance in spite of school absences due to treatments and hospital admissions.

DISCUSSION OF THE RESULTS:

The chronic and recurrent pathology subject to multiple admissions or repetitive consultations, prolonged time-consuming treatments and the vision of inexorable deterioration, create an intense dependence on the environment and especially on the family, which originates a high incidence of psychopathology in patients and their families, especially anxiety, depression and poor social functioning.[37-39]

In the present investigation a total of 14 pediatric patients with Cystic Fibrosis were included, in which it was found that 50% of them were between 9 and 15 years old and half of them were over 15 years old, and no relationship was found between anxiety levels as a trait or as a state with age. A large part (71.43 %) showed anxiety as a trait and the majority (85.72 %) manifested anxiety as a state in medium and high degrees.

Regarding age, we found survival of patients as a result of the integral treatment carried out by the multidisciplinary team, and the evolution in the treatment protocols for these patients, which has managed to reduce mortality in earlier stages of life with respect to previous periods, making it a chronic pathology. A similar situation is described in several studies consulted. [9,14, 18,20]

Gaspar García and collaborators,[18] carried out a study in Spain including patients of all ages with Cystic Fibrosis, and found that 31 % presented anxiety with a higher incidence in older patients. A 21.5 % of CF patients presented depression. Preliminary data from the TIDES study (The International Depression and Anxiety Epidemiological Study) have included CF patients from different international and Spanish centers. They have shown a high prevalence of anxious and/or depressive symptoms in adolescent and adult patients in the United States, Italy, Germany, United Kingdom and Spain and in children and adolescents in Turkey, ranging from 2.1% to 29.4% for depressive symptoms and from 5.6% to 36% for anxious symptoms depending on country, sex or age [41, 43,61] Goldbeck L et al,[62] found that older patients had a higher prevalence of depressive symptoms. Some authors,[60,63] have found that the rate of anxious symptoms has been higher than that of depressive symptoms, results with which we agree.

Studies suggest that the differences in reported prevalences of depression and anxiety are due to various factors that could influence them, including gender, race, marital status, education, employment status, income, household, place of residence, social support, caregiver role, and physical health status as defined by the number of chronic diseases present. For all these reasons, it has been difficult to compare their effects on these mental disorders. [54,59]

Other authors,[44,47,49] have reported a tendency for adolescents with CF to have lower prevalences of depression and anxiety than adults, and good psychological adjustment, with higher levels of anxiety in subjects with a later diagnosis, and even that young adults have similar psychological dynamics to healthy controls. In studies of school-aged children and adolescents with CF,[39,43] have shown a rate of depression ranging from 11% to 14.5%, in contrast to a rate of 2-6% in the general pediatric population. Published rates of anxiety have ranged from 5-9%, which may approximate those of the general pediatric population. These figures are below those found in the present investigation, which we consider to be due to methodological differences in the measurement of anxiety and depression levels.

In adults with CF, rates of depression range from 29% to 46% compared to 5 - 17.5% in the general population and clinically elevated levels of anxiety have been observed in 20.6% of patients compared to 7% of the general population. [28,44,49]

Catastini et al,[64] conducted a longitudinal study in patients with severe CF using the CES-D (Center for Epidemiologic Studies Depression Scale). The results showed that 30% of the patients were above the cut-off point for depression.

The implementation of neonatal screening programs decreases the age of diagnosis. The later the diagnosis is made, the later the initiation of appropriate treatment is delayed, which is associated with increased morbidity and mortality. It is necessary to point out the advantages offered by the Cuban Health System with 100% coverage of maternal and child care, with equal access to health services for the entire population regardless of other demographic or social characteristics, which are cited as limiting factors in early diagnosis in international studies, especially in underdeveloped countries. [29,58]

With respect to the manifestation of depression and anxiety and sex in the CF patients studied, no dependence was found between them; anxiety as a trait with medium intensity predominated in both sexes, although somewhat more in females (42.86%). However, anxiety as a state with high values was manifested more in males than in females, although as was corroborated these differences were not significant.

In the study, depression also had a greater expression in the female sex, but it did not make a significant difference with the male sex.

We consider that one of the reasons limiting the power of the statistical tests in the study is the small sample size, being a disease with a low incidence in the population.

We agree with the results of Gaspar García et al,[18] . These authors found no significant differences in screening scores for depression and anxiety between sexes, although there was a tendency for anxiety scores to be higher in women.

Higher prevalence of depression and anxiety in females with CF compared to males has been reported in the literature,[22,62] although Catastini P. et al,[64] have reflected that not all papers necessarily supported this difference.

When exploring the relationship between the presence of psychopathies in patients with cystic fibrosis and family functioning, in the sample studied there was a significantly higher presence of anxiety as a state in patients with dysfunctional families (35.71%), finding no relationship with anxiety as a trait that presented average values independently of family functioning as well as depression.

Studies consulted have shown high rates of depression in parent caregivers of children with CF when compared to parents of healthy children. [41,57]

In a recent study of parents of children with CF, 28% of parents scored in the clinical range of depression and 37.2% showed symptoms of anxiety. [54] Abbott et al,[53] estimate that a higher percentage of positive screening for depression and anxiety could be related to maladaptive coping strategies ("coping" of the distraction and avoidance types) and explain a poorer perception of quality of life (QoL).

Illán Noguera and collaborators,[65] state that the care of the CF patient implies a supportive approach that is not exclusively focused on the patient, but extends to the entire family, involves a combination of components that may be psychological, social, emotional or clinical, and should be adapted to individual needs.

Wong and Heriot,[66] studied the coping strategies of parents, finding that those who tend to blame themselves or are dismissive of their child's illness experience more distress, anxiety and depression. In this descriptive study, in which 35 parents of children with CF participated, it was also observed that children with CF whose parents have these types of coping behaviors have worse scores on the mental health scale. They further posit that families of chronically ill children tend to be socially isolated. Sometimes parents may decide not to work outside the home in order to provide better care for their sick child. However, it does not seem advisable to adopt this decision, as well as to have few friends and social relations, since it may have a negative influence on the family climate.

Some authors,[50,52] suggest the timely recommendation of routine and standardized annual screening for depression and anxiety in CF patients and their caregivers, as well as the development of decision algorithms for referral and/or treatment by specialized mental health personnel.

According to the severity of the disease in the present study, patients with good and moderate disease status predominated. However, there was no significant association between disease status and the presence of psychopathies. Anxiety as a trait manifested with medium values in most patients regardless of the clinical state of the disease and anxiety as a state between medium and high values. Depression did not show significant differences in the different grades. We also consider that this is due to the small sample size that does not allow us to study the normal behavior of the event.

Gaspar García et al,[18] related the presence of anxiety and depression with older age and worse respiratory status. The presence of depressive and anxious symptoms was associated with worse quality of life. After controlling for demographic (age, sex) and clinical variables (severity according to FEV1), these authors observed that positive screening for depression and anxiety explained a significant percentage of the variance in the health perception domain. In relation to respiratory symptomatology, they only found associations between positive screening for depressive symptoms and desaturation on exertion. In contrast, positive screening for anxious symptoms was associated with worse spirometric parameters (FEV1 less than 50%), presence of desaturation on exertion and worse Bhalla radiological score. These data coincide with those found by Goldbeck L et al,[67] who, when analyzing the association of anxious and depressive symptoms with health status, observed that the presence of hemoptysis or recent pneumothorax was associated with anxiety, while having worse pulmonary function and being on a transplant waiting list were associated with depression. Other studies [21,28, 40,60] have also published significant relationships between depression and anxiety with HRQOL in both the general population and in CF. The levels of self-esteem in CF patients included in the study were not related to the presence of anxiety as a trait, state, or depression, although there was a greater frequency of absence of depression in those with high self-esteem.

It is suggested in the literature that peer relationships promote both the development of appropriate social skills and the acquisition of a healthy self-concept. Friends are a source of support for children with CF, allowing them to minimize their visible differences from others. However, a chronic illness such as this can also increase vulnerability in peer interactions.[68]

Adolescents with CF may also choose non-adherent behaviors when experiencing peer pressure in social situations. [49,65]

A study by Brengballe et al, comparing the well-being of 43 children with CF aged 7-14 years with that of a sample of 1121 healthy children noted that behavioral problems in these adolescents are often seen as responses to anxiety and stress. Peer acceptance, or lack thereof, can be especially painful for the entire family, insofar as the child feels rejected and isolated, which in turn can contribute to stress and deterioration of the family climate. [69]

Harrop M,[70] found that children with CF do not differ from the group of healthy children in depression, self-concept and disruptive behavior, although they did score higher on the anxiety scale. Young people with CF are less developed in social relationships and sexuality, have delayed puberty and are shorter in stature, which implies some isolation from peer groups.

It is suggested that the higher levels of depression among chronically ill adolescents may not be due to inherent psychopathological factors, but rather to a reaction to the limits imposed by the family and society, implying that this situation is preventable. The adolescent's ability to achieve independence depends, to some extent, on the support received from the family.[65]

On the social level, adolescents in particular have difficulties in establishing relationships with other people and sometimes express feelings of isolation and loneliness.

According to research by the Spanish Federation against Cystic Fibrosis presented in its manual of protective measures for family members of people with CF, Cuidarme Bien para Cuidar Mejor, in 71.14% of cases with CF, it is the mother who assumes the main role of caregiver. While the father works and/or stays a bit more on the sidelines of the disease. As a result of this, multiple factors may arise that can directly affect the patient's emotional, physical, mental, work and social state, among others.[71]

Dr. Morey in the integral analysis of all the indicators of the free and family drawings found that 29.5 % presented with immaturity, fixed ideas or worries, anxiety and impulsivity, preoccupation with the disease and in the relationship with maternal and paternal figures. They also express that most of the patients in the study, without specifying whether or not they reach parameterized clinical psychiatric diagnoses, present affectations in the emotional plane referred to themselves or to the family environment, predominating in them environmental tension and insecurity, inhibition of the emotional response and anguish with dysphoria, which proves the usefulness of its use as part of the diagnostic process for revealing all the richness of their subjectivity and hence its value in terms of the latent content of their environment.[46]

Mónica Cebrián Pinar found in a comparative quality of life study that when people with CF have been compared to healthy people, overall QOL results have shown that, generally, adults with CF have an equal or better overall QOL than control subjects (e.g., satisfaction with broader dimensions of life, such as independence, work, relationships, and family); however, subjects with lower lung function (FEV1 < 30% predicted) report lower overall QOL.[60]

Triangulation

The results of the anxiety, depression and self-esteem assessment instruments showed greater affectation of these spheres in patients where family dysfunction and difficulties in the emotional control of parents and caregivers were identified, which was the fundamental reason that generates stress and especially anxiety in these patients. Although in the statistical analyses the relationship of these associations could not be corroborated.

CONCLUSIONS:

Patients with Cystic Fibrosis were mainly of school age, especially adolescents with a slight predominance of the female sex, although these demographic characteristics were not related to the presence of affective symptoms. Medium values of anxiety as a trait and medium to high values of anxiety as a state were frequent, with a predominance of patients without depression or with mild depression, although this was slightly more frequent in the female sex. In dysfunctional families, there was evidence of high levels of anxiety as a state in the patients, and no relationship was found between affective symptoms and the severity of the disease, or with self-esteem. The qualitative analysis identified that dysfunctional families, with difficulties in coping with the disease, generated higher levels of anxiety in the patient and difficulties with self-esteem, although not with the evolution of the disease. Most of the patients were affected in the personal, family and social areas, and several areas of conflict were affected.

RECOMMENDATIONS:

- Conduct intervention research aimed at achieving adequate family, school and social management of patients with Cystic Fibrosis.
- Conduct longitudinal cohort studies to assess the patient's psychoaffective state during the evolution of the disease and the response to follow-up and psychological treatment.

BIBLIOGRAPHIC REFERENCES:

1.	Aliño Pellicer SF, Antelo Landeira MC, Baamonde Vidarte A, Beltrán Bengoechea B, Berná Torres N, Calvo Medina V. White Paper on Cystic Fibrosis care [Internet]. Valencia: Spanish Federation against Cystic Fibrosis; 2010.	Availableat: http://www.fqasturias.org/ver.aspx?id=26.

2.	Red CM. Cystic fibrosis or mucoviscidosis. In: Torre ME, Pelayo GE. Pediatrics. Havana: Editorial Ciencias Médicas; 2007.p.1012-55.

3.	del Campo Avilés J A. Electrolytes in sweat. CCM [Internet]. 2013 [cited

24 Feb 2014];	17 (3).	Availablefrom:

http://scielo.sld.cu/scielo.php?script=sci_serial&pid=1560-

4381&lng=en&nrm=iso

4.	Castaños C, Rentería F. National consensus on cystic fibrosis. Arch Argent Pediatr [Internet]. 2008 [cited 24 Feb 2014]; 106(5). Available from:

http://.sap.org.ar/docs/profesionales/consensos/v106n5a12e.pdf

5.	Vaglio A, Pizzo L, Quadrelli A, Gueçaimburú R, Pagano S, Quadrelli R. Limitations of molecular genetic studies in the diagnostic process of cystic fibrosis. Rev. Méd. Urug. [Internet]. 2011 [cited 12 Jan 2015], 27(3): [approx. 8 p.]. Available from:

http://www.scielo.edu.uy/scielo.php?script=sci_pdf&pid=S0303-

32952011000300002&lng=en&nrm=iso&tlng=en.

6.	Accurso FJ. Cystic Fibrosis. In: Goldman L, Schafer AI. Goldman's Cecil Medicine. 24th ed [Internet]. Philadelphia: Saunders Elsevier; 2012. p. 544-

548. Disponible en:

https://www.clinicalkey.com/#!/ContentPlayerCtrl/doPlayContent/3-s2.0-

B9781437716047000890/{%22scope%22:%22all%22,%22query%22:%22C

ystic%20Fibrosis%22}

7.	Cohen-Cymberknoh M, Shoseyov D, Kerem E. Managing Cystic

Fibrosis. Am. J. Respir. Crit. Care Med [Internet]. 2011 [cited 15 Feb 2012]; 183(11): [approx. 8 p.]. Available from: http://www.atsjournals.org/doi/full/10.1164/rccm.201009-1478CI.

8.   Royce FH, Carl JC. Health-related quality of life in cystic fibrosis. Curr Opin Pediatr [Internet]. 2011 [cited 15 Feb 2012]; 23. Available from: http://www.ncbi.nlm.nih.gov/pubmed/21900781

9.   Antonelli Cohen M, Gonçalves de Oliveira Ribeiro MA, Fernando Ribeiro A, Ribeiro JD, Moreno Morcillo A. Quality of life assessment in patients with cystic fibrosis by means of the Cystic Fibrosis Questionnaire. J Bras Pneumol [Internet]. 2011 [cited 28 Jan 2014]; 37(2): [approx. 8 p.]. Available from: http://www.scielo.br/pdf/jbpneu/v37n2/en_v37n2a08.pdf.

10.   Davis SD, Ferkol T. Identifying the Origins of Cystic Fibrosis Lung Disease. NEJM [Internet]. 2013 [cited 28 Jan 2014]; 368 (21). Available from: http://www.nejm.org/doi/pdf/10.1056/NEJMe1303487

11.   Meyer P, Lazarte G, Zamora G, Tanuz H, Figueroa Turienzo J. 38th Argentine Congress of Respiratory Medicine Argentine Association of Respiratory Medicine: epidemiological and genetic data of patients with cystic fibrosis in the province of Jujuy-Argentina. Rev Am Med Resp [Internet]. 2010 [cited 28 Jan 2014]. Available from: http://www.ramr.org.ar/articulos/suplemento_38_congreso/sup_38c_trabajos_libres.pdf

12.   Cystic Fibrosis Foundation. Patient Registry. In: Annual Data Report [Internet]. Bethesda, Maryland: Cystic Fibrosis Foundation; 2012 [cited 28 Jan2014]. Available. From: http://www.cff.org/UploadedFiles/research/ClinicalResearch/PatientRegistry Report/2012-CFF-Patient-Registry.pdf.

13.   Salcedo A, Gartner S, Girón RM, García MD. LACK OF CHAPTER. In: Tratado de fibrosis quística [Internet]. Madrid: Justim; 2012 [cited 28 Jan

2014]. Available from:
http://www.aeped.es/sites/default/files/documentos/tratado_fibro_quistica.pd f

14.   Guzmán Pileta K, Del Campo Mulet E, Nápoles Smith N, Toledano Grave de Peralta   Y   ,   Coello   Morales   D . Main clinical and epidemiological characteristics of patients with cystic fibrosis in the province of Santiago de Cuba.   clinicoepidemiological characteristics of patients with cystic fibrosis in the province of Santiago de Cuba. MEDISAN [Internet]. 2011 Feb [cited30 Aug 2016]; 15(2).   Available   en: http://scielo.sld.cu/scielo.php?script=sci_arttext&pid=S1029-30192011000200002&lng=es.

15.   Pereyro S, Renteria F, Fernando V, Nadeo J, Paba P, Inwentarz S, Laura B. Guidelines for the diagnosis and treatment of patients with cystic fibrosis. Update[Internet].   2014   [cited   28   Jan   2014].   Available   from: http://www.sap.org.ar/docs/profesionales/consensos/consenso_fq_2014.pdf

16.   Duran-Palomino D. Compliance with British Thoracic Society respiratory rehabilitation recommendations in patients with Cystic Fibrosis: a study in Colombian physiotherapists. Rev Peru Med Exp Salud Publica [Internet]   2013   [cited28Jan2014   ], 30(2).   Availablefrom: http://www.scielo.org.pe/scielo.php?script=sci_arttext&pid=S1726-46342013000200016

17.   Haack A, CG. Multidisciplinary care in cystic fibrosis: a clinical-nutrition review. Nutr. Hosp [Internet]. 2012 [cited 28 Jan 2014]. (2). Available from: https://www.ncbi.nlm.nih.gov/pubmed/22732957

18.   Gaspar García I, Olveira Fuster C, Espíldora Hernández F, Jimeno Galván R, Dorado Galindo A, Olveira Fuster G. Depressive and anxious symptoms in patients with cystic fibrosis: influence on health-related quality of

life. Rev. Esp. Torac [Internet]. 2012 [cited 2 Jun 2016]; 24(2). Available. at:

http://www.neumosur.net/files/1.%20ORIGINAL%2024-2.pdf

19.	Gil B, Ballester R, Gómez S, Abizanda R. Emotional affect of patients admitted to an intensive care unit. Journal of Psychopathology and Clinical Psychology [Internet]. 2013 [cited 2 Jun 2016]; 18(2). Available from:

http://www.revistas.uned.es/index.php/RPPC/article/download/12769/pdf_5

20.	Castillo Izquierdo GC, Lozano Pérez T, García Sánchez JB. Emotional disorders in children and adolescents with cystic fibrosis. Rev. Hosp. Psychiatric Havana [Internet]. 2013 [cited 2 Jun 2016]; 10(1). Available from:

http://www.revistahph.sld.cu/hph0113/hph09113.html

21.	Quintana-Gallego E. Cystic fibrosis: association between depression, anxiety and health-related quality of life. Rev Esp Patol Torac [Internet]. 2012 [cited 2 Jun 2016]; 24 (2). Available from:

http://www.neumosur.net/files/EDITORIAL%2024-2.pdf

22.	Modi AC, Driscoll KA, Montag-leifing K, Acton JD. Screening for symptoms of depression and anxiety in adolescents and young adults with cystic fibrosis. Ped Pulmonol [Internet]. 2011 [cited 24 Feb 2016]; 46. Available from:

https://www.ncbi.nlm.nih.gov/pmc/articles/PMC3462584/pdf/nihms291565. pdf

23.	Helms SW, Dellon EP, Prinstein MJ. Friendship quality and health? Related outcomes among adolescents with cystic fibrosis. Journal of Pediatric Psychology [Internet]. 2015 [cited 2 Jun 2016]; 40(3). Available from:

http://jpepsy.oxfordjournals.org/content/40/3/349.full.pdf+html

24.	Ernst MM, Johnson MC,Stark LJ. Developmental and psychosocial issues in cystic fibrosis. Child Adolesc Psychiatric Clin N Am [Internet]. 2010 [cited

2 Jun 2016]; 19(2). Availablefrom:

http://www.ncbi.nlm.nih.gov/pmc/articles/PMC2874200/

25.	Kopp BT, Hayes D, Ghera P, Patel A, Kirkby S, Kowatch RA, Splaingard

M. Pilot trial of light therapy for depression in hospitalized patients with cystic fibrosis. Journal of Affective Disorders [Internet]. 2016 [cited 2 Jun 2016]; 189. Available from: http://www.jad-journal.com/article/S0165-0327%2815%2930574-7/pdf.

26.   Garcia G, Oliva M, Smith BA. Survey of collaborative mental health providers in cystic fibrosis centers in the United States. General Hospital Psychiatry [Internet].2015 [cited 2 Jun 2016]; 37. Available from: http://www.sciencedirect.com/science/article/pii/S0163834315000493

27.   Sly PD, Gangell CL, Chen L, Ware RS, Ranganathan S, Mott LS, et al. Risk Factors for Bronchiectasis in Children with Cystic Fibrosis. NEJM [Internet]. 2013 [cited January 2014]; 368(21). Available from: http://www.nejm.org/doi/pdf/10.1056/NEJMoa1301725

28.   Gómez Poo A. Influence of respiratory physiotherapy on quality of life in adolescents and adults with cystic fibrosis [Thesis]. Spain: Gimbernat-Cantabria University School (Torrelavega); 2014 [cited 2 Jun 2016]. Available from: http://repositorio.unican.es/xmlui/bitstream/handle/10902/6047/G%C3%93 MEZ%20POO,%20%C3%81ngela.pdf?sequence=1

29.   Ministry of Health. National Cystic Fibrosis Program: Technical Programmatic Guidelines for Diagnosis   and Treatment [Internet]. Colombia: Ministry of Health; 2012 [cited 12 Jul 2016]. Available from: http://respiratorio.minsal.cl/pdf/fibrosis/adulto/guia_clinica_fq_2012.pdf

30.   Davis SD, Ferkol T. Identifying the Origins of Cystic Fibrosis Lung Disease. NEJM [Internet]. May 2013 [cited 12 Jul 2016] ; 368(21). Available from: http://www.nejm.org/doi/pdf/10.1056/NEJMe1303487

31.   Akabas MH. Cystic fibrosis transmembrane conductance regulator. Structure and function of an epithelial chloride channel. J. Biol. Chem [Internet]. 2000 [cited 2013 Mar 15]; 275(6). Available from: http://www.jbc.org/content/275/6/3729.long

32.   Navarro H, Kolbach M, Repetto G, Guiraldes E, Harris P, Foradori A, et al. Genotype-phenotype correlation in a group of patients with cystic fibrosis. Rev. med. chile [Internet]. 2002 [cited 15 March 2013]; 130(5). Available from: http://www.scielo.cl/scielo.php?script=sci_arttext&pid=S0034-98872002000500001

33.   D'AlessandroV , RenteríaF , FernándezA , MartínezMI   , Segal   E. Comparison of clinical-functional status in children with cystic fibrosis detected by neonatal screening or clinical symptoms. Arch Argent Pediatr [Internet]. 2009 [cited 15 March 2013]; 107(5). Available from: http://www.scielo.org.ar/scielo.php?script=sci_arttext&pid=S0325-00752009000500010

34.   Fuentes Fernández G, Abreu Suárez G, Pérez Brunet AP, González Valdés JA, Portuondo Leyva R. Characterization of cystic fibrosis in the first year of life. Cuban Journal of Pediatrics [Internet]. 2014 [cited 2 Jun 2016]; 86(4). Available from: http://scielo.sld.cu/pdf/ped/v86n4/ped03414.pdf 35.Bryant JM, Grogono DM, Greaves D, Foweraker J, Roddick I, Inns T.   Whole-genomesequencing to identify transmission of Mycobacterium abscessus among patients with cystic fibrosis: a retrospective cohort study.

Lancet [Internet]. 2013 [cited 2 Jun 2016]; 381(9877): [approx. 9 p.]. Available from:

http://www.ncbi.nlm.nih.gov/pmc/articles/PMC3664974/?tool=pubmed

36.Smith BA, Cogswell A, Garcia G. Vitamin D and depressive symptoms in Children with cystic fibrosis. Psychosomatics [Internet]. 2014 [cited 2 Jun 2016]; (1). Available   From:

http://www.sciencedirect.com/science/article/pii/S0033318213000133

37.Carter BR, Wray JR, Red NS. The chronically in child and family illness. Family developmental perspective on cystic fibrosis. Psychosomatic fall [Internet]. 2008   [cited2jun2016   ];   33(4).   Available   from:

https://www.researchgate.net/publication/21693684_The_chronically_ill_chi

ld_and_family_stress_Family_development_perspectives_on_cystic_fibrosis

38.WHO. Noncommunicable diseases and mental health. Chronic diseases and health promotion. Preparing health care professionals for the 21st century. The challenge of chronic diseases. Switzerland: WHO;

2005. p 15

39.   Williams SB, O'Connor EA, Eder M, Whitlock EP. Screening for child and adolescent depression in primary care settings: a systematic evidence review for the US Preventive Services Task Force. Pediatrics [Internet]. 2009 [cited 2 Jun 2016]; 123(4). Available from: http://pediatrics.aappublications.org/content/123/4/e716

40.   Suárez Soto E. Quality of life and family functioning in adolescents with depression in public health centers [Thesis]. Santiago, Chile: University of Chile; 2013 [cited 18 Mar 2016]. Available from: http://repositorio.uchile.cl/bitstream/handle/2250/130104/TESIS%20FINAL.pdf?sequence=1

41.   Quittner AL, Goldbeck L, Abbott J, Duff A, Lambrecht P, Solé A, et al. Prevalence of depression and anxiety in patients with cystic fibrosis and parent caregivers: results of The International Depression Epidemiological Study across nine countries. Thorax [Internet]. 2014 [cited 18 Mar 2016];

69.   Available at: http://thorax.bmj.com/content/69/12/1090.full.pdf+html

42.Kendler KS, Myers J, Prescott CA. Sex differences in the relationship between social support and risk for major depression: a longitudinal study of opposite-sex twin pairs. Am J Psychiatry [Internet]. 2005 [cited 2 Jun 2016]; 162(2). Available. Available from: https://www.ncbi.nlm.nih.gov/pubmed/15677587

43.   Besier T, Goldbeck L. Anxiety and depression in adolescents with CF and their caregivers. Journal of Cystic Fibrosis [Internet]. 2011 [cited 24 Feb 2013]; 10. Available from: http://ac.els-cdn.com/S1569199311001214/1-s2.0-S1569199311001214-main.pdf?_tid=2f3d6834-647d-11e6-a897-

00000aacb362&acdnat=1471440130_1782bd19510d9a82b3e4672553ba72b_b

44.   Habib AR, Manji J, Wilcox PG, Javer AR, Buxton JA, Quon BS. A Systematic Review of Factors Associated with Health-Related Quality of Life in Adolescents and Adults with Cystic Fibrosis. Ann Am Thorac Soc [Internet]. 2015 [cited 18 Mar 2016]; 12(3). Available from: http://www.atsjournals.org/doi/pdf/10.1513/AnnalsATS.201408-393OC

45.   Bones Rocha K, Forns Serrallonga D, Chamarro Lusar A. Relationship between Treatment Adherence, Family Climate and Educational Styles. R. Interam. Psychol [Internet]. 2009 [cited 24 Feb 2013]; 43(2). Available from: http://pepsic.bvsalud.org/pdf/rip/v43n2/v43n2a15.pdf

46.   Castillo Izquierdo GC, Lozano Pérez L. Free and family drawing for the diagnosis of emotional disorders in patients with Cystic Fibrosis.

Rev. Havana Psychiatric Hospital [Internet]. 2012 [cited 2 Jun 2016], 9(3). Available   from: http://www.revistahph.sld.cu/Revista%203-2012/hph05312.html.

47.   De Maso DR, Martini DR, CAhen LA. Practice parameter for the psychiatric assessment and management of physically ill children and adolescents. J. Am. Acad. Child Adolesc. Psychiatry. 2009 [cited 2 Jun 2016]; 48(2).   Available   from: http://www.jaacap.com/article/S0890-8567%2809%2960019- 8/pdf

48.   Girón RM, Cuadrado F. Psychological aspects of the patient with cystic fibrosis: what happens when the disease progresses? Rev Patol Respir [Internet]. 2006   [cited   2013   Mar   15];   9(2).   Available   from: http://www.revistadepatologiarespiratoria.org/descargas/pr_9-2_53-54.pdf

49.   Casier A, Goubert L, Theunis M, Huse D, De Baets F, Matthys D, Crombez

G. Acceptance and well-being in adolescents and young adults with cystic

fibrosis: a prospective study. J Pediatr Psychol [Internet]. 2011 [cited 18 Mar 2016]; 36. Available from:http://jpepsy.oxfordjournals.org/content/36/4/476.full.pdf+html

50.   Spanish Federation of Cystic Fibrosis. Emotional impact [Internet]. Valencia, Spain: Spanish Federation of Cystic Fibrosis; 2015 [cited 12 Jul 2016]. Available from: http://www.fibrosisquistica.org/pdf/impacto_emocional.pdf.

51.   Driscoll KA, Johnson SB, Barker D, Quittner AL, Deeb LC, Geller DE, Gondor M, Silverstein JH. Risk factors associated with depressive symptoms in caregivers of children with type 1 diabetes or cystic fibrosis. J Pediatr Psychol [Internet]. 2011 Sep [cited 24 Feb 2013]; 35(8). Available from: https://www.ncbi.nlm.nih.gov/pubmed/20097908

52.   Sawicki GS, Rasouliyan L, McMullen AH, Wagener JS, McColley SA, Pasta DJ, Quittner AL. Longitudinal assessment of health-related quality of life in an observational cohort of patients with cystic fibrosis. Pediatr Pulmonol [Internet]. 2011 [cited 24 Feb 2013]; 46(1). Available from: https://www.ncbi.nlm.nih.gov/pubmed/20848580

53.   Abbott J, Hurley MA, Morton AM, Conway SP. Longitudinal association between lung function and health-related quality of life in cystic fibrosis. Thorax [Internet]. 2013 [cited 18 Feb 2015]; 68(2). Available from: https://www.ncbi.nlm.nih.gov/pubmed/23143792

54.   Abbott J, Morton AM, Hurley MA, Conway SP. Longitudinal impact of demographic and clinical variables on health-related quality of life in cystic fibrosis. BMJ Open [Internet]. 2015 [cited 25 March 2016]; 5(5). Available from: http://bmjopen.bmj.com/content/5/5/e007418.abstract

55.   Feltrim MI, Coelho AA, Scatimburgo MM, Pereira GM, Pego-Fernandes P. Quality of life assessment in two consecutive years of patients in a waiting list for lung transplantation. Transplant Proc [Internet]. 2014 Nov [cited 25 March 2016];   46(9). Available at: https://www.ncbi.nlm.nih.gov/pubmed/25420822

56.   Barrio Gómez de Agüero MI, García Hernández G, Gartner S, Cystic Fibrosis Working Group. Protocol for diagnosis and follow-up of patients with

cystic fibrosis. An Pediatr (Barc) [Internet]. 2009 [cited September 2012]; 71(3). Available from: http://www.sefq.es/ProtocSENP09.pdf

57.   Dunst C J, Trivette C, Deal A. Enabling and empowering families: Principles and guidelines for practice. Cambridge: USA: Brookline Book, Inc; 1988.

58.   Olivo Pallo PA. Correlation of spirometric values with the Shwachman clinical score and the Brasfield radiological score, in the evaluation of patients with a diagnosis of Cystic Fibrosis, seen in the outpatient clinic of the Pneumology service of the Eugenio Espejo specialty hospital in the city of Quito, in the period June-August 2014 [Thesis]. Quito, Ecuador: Universidad Central; 2015   [cited   24   Feb   2013]. http://www.dspace.uce.edu.ec/bitstream/25000/4700/1/T-UCE-0006- 103.pdf.

59.   Fuentes Fernández G, Portuondo Leyva R. Characterization of fibrocystic patients who died during the course of their disease. Centro Habana Pediatric Hospital, 1993-2012 [Thesis]. Centro Habana: Hospital Docente Centro Habana; 2013.

60.   Cebrián Pinar M. Cystic fibrosis. Comparison of three quality of life questionnaires [Thesis]. Valencia, Spain: University of Valencia; 2015 [cited2 Jun 2016]. Available from: http://mobiroderic.uv.es/bitstream/handle/10550/50908/Tesis%20Doctoral% 20M%C3%B3nica%20Cebri%C3%A1n%202015.pdf?sequence=1&isAllow ed=y.

61.   Quittner AL, Cruz I, Blackwell LS, Schechter MS. The International Depression and Anxiety Epidemiological Stude (TIDES): preliminary results from the United States. J Cyst Fibros [Internet]. 2011 [cited 2016 Mar 25]; 9 (Suppl1). Availablefrom: http://www.cysticfibrosisjournal.com/article/S1569-1993(10)60366-9/pdf.

62.   Goldbeck L, Besier T, Hinz A, Singer S, Quittner AL and the TIDES study group. Prevalence of symptoms of anxiety and depression in German

patients with cystic fibrosis. Chest [Internet]. 2011 [cited 25 March 2016]; 138. Available at: https://www.ncbi.nlm.nih.gov/pubmed/20472857

63.   Olveira C, Sole A, Girón RM, Quintana-Gallego E, Mondejar P, Baranda F, et al. Depression and anxiety symptoms in Spanish adult patients with cystic fibrosis: associations with health-related quality of life. Gen Hosp Psychiatry [Internet]. 2016 [cited 12 June 2016]; 40. Available from: https://www.ncbi.nlm.nih.gov/pubmed/26971246

64.   Catastini P, Festini F, Di Marco S, Genovese C, Grande A, Iacinti E, et al. The International Depression and Anxiety Epidemiological Study (TIDES): results from Italy. J Cyst Fibros [Internet]. 2011 [cited 25 March 2016]; 9 (Suppl1).   Available   at: http://www.cysticfibrosisjournal.com/article/S1569-1993(10)60366-9/pdf.

65.   Illán Noguera CR, del Camino Álvarez Martínez M, Martínez Rabadán M, Pina Díaz LM, Guillén Pérez F, Bernal Barquero M, García Díaz S, García Díaz MJ. Nursing care and counseling in children and adolescents with cystic fibrosis: a literature review. Revista Enfermería Docente [Internet].2014 [cited 2 Jun   2016];   1(102).   Available   from: http://www.revistaenfermeriadocente.es/index.php/ENDO/article/view/3/pdf _2

66.   Wong MG, Heriot SA. Parents of children with cystic fibrosis: how they hope, cope and despair. Child Care, Health Dev [Internet]. 2008 [cited 2 Jun 2016]; 34(3). Available from:

67.   Goldbeck L, Besier T, Hinz A, Singer S, Quittner AL and the TIDES study group. Prevalence of symptoms of anxiety and depression in German patients with cystic fibrosis. Chest [Internet]. 2010 [cited 2 Jun 2016]; 138. Available from: http://www.ncbi.nlm.nih.gov/pubmed/20472857

68.   Fernández Rodríguez M, Martin Muñoz P. Perceived quality of life in children with cystic fibrosis is worse in the group aged 8 to 12 years. Control in hospital versus follow-up in peripheral centers offered few differences Evidencias

en Pediatría [Internet]. 2006 [cited 2013 Mar 15]; 2(3). Available from:
http://riberdis.cedd.net/bitstream/handle/11181/4319/Lacalidaddevidapercibi
daporni%C3%B1osconfibrosis.pdf?sequence=1&rd=0031659348271634

69.   Brengballe V, Thastum M, Schiotz PO. Psychosocial problems in children with cystic fibrosis. Acta Paediatr [Internet]. 2007 [cited 15 March 2013];

96. Available at: http://www.ncbi.nlm.nih.gov/pubmed/17187605 70.Harrop M, Psychosocial impact of cystic fibrosis in adolescence. Paediatr

Nurs [Internet]. 2007 [cited 2013 Mar 15]; 19(10). Available from:

http://journals.rcni.com/doi/pdfplus/10.7748/paed2007.12.19.10.41.c6432

71.   Espinosa Godoy MT, Trejo Valdivia KP. Intervention in a case of Cystic Fibrosis [Thesis]. Barcelona: ISEP; 2013 [cited 2013 March 15]. Available from:

http://www.isep.es/tesina/intervencion-en-un-caso-de-fibrosis-quistica/

APPENDIX . Trait-State Anxiety Inventory for Children

IDAREN

Name and surname:_____ -:_____________________

Age:_______Sex: -School: -_____________________

Grade:_______________M unicipality: -___- Date:_____/_____/-

PART ONE

In the first part you will find a phrase used to say something about yourself. Read each phrase and point to the answer that says **HOW YOU FEEL RIGHT NOW**, at this moment. There are no good or bad answers. Don't dwell too long on each sentence and answer by pointing to the answer that best says how you feel RIGHT NOW.

	Nothing	Something	Much
I feel calm			
2. I feel restless			
I feel nervous			
4. I feel rested			
5. I am afraid			
6. I am relaxed			
7. I am worried			
8. I am satisfied			
9. I feel happy			
10.I feel safe			
11.I feel well			
12.I feel annoyed			
13.I feel pleasantly			
14.I am frightened			
15.I am confused			
16.I feel encouraged			
17.I feel distressed			
18.I feel cheerful			
19.I feel disgruntled			

20. I feel sad			

INSTRUCTIONS

PART TWO (IDAREN for Children)

In the second part you will find more sentences to say something about yourself. Read each sentence and point to the answer that says how you **FEEL in GENERAL**, not just at this moment. There are no bad or good answers. Don't dwell too long on each sentence and answer by pointing to the answers that best say how you feel **OVERALL.**

	Almost Never	Something	A Often
1. I worry about making mistakes			
2. I feel like crying			
3. I feel unhappy			
4. I find it difficult to make a decision			
5. I find it hard to face my problems			
6. I worry too much			
7. I find myself annoyed			
8. Unimportant thoughts pop into my head and bother me.			
9. I worry about things at school			
10.I find it hard to decide what to do			
11.I notice that my heart beats faster.			
12.Although I don't say it, I am afraid			

13.I worry about things that may happen.			
14.I find it hard to fall asleep at night.			
15.I have strange sensations in the stomach			
16.I am concerned about what others think of me.			
17.I am so influenced by the problems that I do not I can forget them for a while			
18.I take things too seriously			
19.I find many difficulties in my life			
20.I feel less happy than other kids.			

Zung and Count test	Very few times	Sometimes	Many times	Always
1-I feel sad or depressed	1	2	3	4
2-In the mornings I feel better than in the mornings. in the afternoons	4	3	2	1
3-Frequently I feel like cry and sometimes I cry	1	2	3	4
4-I have a hard time sleeping or I sleep poorly at night	1	2	3	4
5-I now have as much appetite as before.	4	3	2	1
6-I'm still attracted to the opposite sex	4	3	2	1
7-I think I am losing weight	1	2	3	4
8-I am constipated	1	2	3	4
9-I have palpitations	1	2	3	4
10- Anything makes me tired	1	2	3	4
11-My head is as clear as formerly	4	3	2	1
12- I do things with the same ease from before	4	3	2	1

13- I feel agitated or uneasy, no I can stand still	1	2	3	4
14-I have confidence and hope in the future	4	3	2	1
15- I feel more irritable than usually	1	2	3	4
16-Decision making meeting	4	3	2	1
17-I believe I am useful and necessary for the people	4	3	2	1
18-A pleasant encounter to live	4	3	2	1
19- It would be better if I died for the others	1	2	3	4
20- I like the same things that I usually liked them	4	3	2	1

ANNEX 4. Answer the following table by marking the answer with an x:

Explanatory note for answering:

Almost never: Refers to an action that almost never occurs.

Rarely: Refers to an action that occurs less frequently and sporadically.

Sometimes: Refers to an action that occurs sporadically.

Often: Refers to an action that is performed more frequently. Almost always:

Refers to an action that is performed on a regular basis.

Table 1.

Below is a group of situations that may or may not occur in your family, You must classify and mark with an X your answer, according to the frequency in which the situation arises.

		Almost never	Few times	A times	Many times	Almost always
1	Decisions are made for important family matters.					
2	Harmony prevails in my house.					
3	In my house everyone fulfills their responsibilities.					
4	Manifestations of affection are part of our daily lives.					
5	We express ourselves without insinuations, in a clear and straightforward manner.					
6	We can accept the shortcomings of others and cope with them.					
7	We take into consideration					

	experiences of other families, in the face of difficult situations.					
8	When someone in the family has a problem, others help them.					
9	Tasks are distributed as follows that no one is overloaded.					

10	Family customs can be modified in the face of certain situations.					
11	We can discuss various topics without fear.					
12	When faced with a difficult family situation, we are able to seek help from other people.					
13	The interests and needs of each individual are respected by the core family.					
14	We show each other the love we have for each other we have.					

ANNEX 5. MEDICAL HISTORY REVIEW GUIDE.

Patient's name:___________________________________ Age:

___________________ Sex:________HC:__________

Shwachman Score:

Grade	Pts	Activity general	Exploration physics	Nutrition	Radiology

Excellent 25	(86-100)	Full general activity; plays ball, attends school regularly, etc.	Normal; no coughing; pulse and respirations normal; lungs clear; posture adequate.	Maintains weight and size > P25;well-modeled stool; muscle mass and tonus normal.	Clean lung fields.
Good 20	(71-85)	Lacks stamina and is tired at the end of the day; good school attendance.	Normal resting pulse and respirations; infrequent cough and throat clearing; no digital deformity; lungs clear; emphysema minimum.	Weight and size between P10 and P25; slightly abnormal stools; adequate muscle tone and mass.	Minimal thickening of bronchovascular images; emphysema begins.

Slight 15	(56-70)	Voluntarily rests during the day; tires easily after exertion; irregular school attendance.	Coughing occasionally in the morning on rising; respirations are slightly mild, mild emphysema; noisy breathing; rarely localized stitches; starts drumstick deformity of the digits.	Weight and size between P3 and P10; stoolsgenerally abnormal, abundant and poorly molded; little, if any, abdominal distention; decreased muscle tone and masses.	Mild emphysema with patchy atelectasis; increased bronchovascular imaging
Moderate 10	(41-55)	Receives classes at home; dyspneic after a cortopaseo; rests a lot.	Frequent and usually productive cough; moderate emphysema; there may be	Weight and size < P3; poorly molded, abundant feces, fats and foul smells	Moderate emphysema; diffuse areas of atelectasis with suggestive overlapping areas deinfection;

			thoracic deformity; frequent rales; acropacities; acropaquias ++/+++.	flaccid nodules and decreased muscle masses; dominal distensionb mild to moderate.	minimal bronchial dilatation .
Severe 5	(< 41)	Orthopneic; limited to bed or chair.	Very frequent coughing on access; tachypnea; tachycardia; significant pulmonary changes; signs of cardiac insufficiency; acropacities++. +/++++.	Significant malnutrition; severe thing rectal prolapse; fatty, foul-smelling, frequent and abundant stools.	Extensive alterations due to obstruction and infection; lobar atelectasis and bronchiectasis.

Severity of the disease in the patient:_______________________________

ANNEX 6. SELF-ESTEEM QUESTIONNAIRE

Central University of Las Villas Faculty of Psychology

Name:____ Age:_

____

Read carefully the following sentences and answer YES or NO according to the relation in which what is expressed corresponds to you. There are no good or bad answers, it is about knowing what is your situation with the issue raised.

Proposals	Yes	No
1-People's problems affect me very little.		
2-I have trouble speaking in public.		
3-I would change many things about myself if I could.		
4-I can easily make a decision.		
5-I am a nice person.		
6-I get angry easily at home.		
7- I have a hard time getting used to something new.		
8- I am a popular person among people my age.		
9- My family generally takes my feelings into account.		
10-I give up easily		
11-My family expects a lot from me.		
12-I find it hard to accept myself as I am		
13-My life is very complicated		

14-My colleagues almost always accept my ideas.		
15-I have a low opinion of myself		
16-Many times I would like to leave home		
17-I often feel uncomfortable in my job.		
18-I am less handsome (or pretty) than most people.		
19-If I have something to say, I generally say it.		
20-My family understands me		
21- Others are better accepted than me		
22-I feel pressure from my family		
23-I often get discouraged with what I am doing.		
24-Many times I would like to be someone else		
25- I can be trusted very little		

ANNEX 7.SENTENCE COMPLETION TEST (ROTTER)

Name and surname: Age_________________________ Sex:_______

Schooling _Marital status________________Occupation and place of work or study_

____

____

-Test Instructions: Complete or finish these sentences to express your true feelings, ideas or opinions.

Try to complete all the sentences:

1.   I like____

2.   The happiest time

____

3.   I would like to know

____

4.   At home

____

5.   Sorry

____

6.   At bedtime

____

7.   Men

____

8.   The best

____

9.   It bothers me

____

10.   People

____

11.   A mother

____

12.   Sorry

____

13.   My greatest fear

-

____

—

14.At school

-

____

—

15.I cannot

-

____

—

16.Sports

____

17.When I was a boy (or girl)

-

____

—

18.My nerves

____

19.   Other people

____

20.   Suffer

-

____

____

21.I failed

____

23.   My mind

____

24.   The sexual impulse

____

25.   My future

____

26.   I need

____

27.   Marriage

____

28.   I am better when

____

29.   Sometimes

____

30.   I am in pain

____

31.   I hate

____

32.   This place

____

33.   I am very

____

34.   The main concern

35.   Desire

36.   My father

____

37.   I secretly

____

38.   I

____

Divisions

____

40.   My biggest problem is

____

41.   The majority of women

____

42.   The work

____

43.   Master

____

44.   Makes me nervous

____

45.   My main ambition

____

46.   I prefer

____

47.   My main problem in choosing a career, profession or job

48.   I would like to be

____

49.

49.   I think my best skills are

____

50.   My personality

____

51.   Happiness

____

ANNEX 8. IPJ (INVENTORY OF YOUTH PROBLEMS)

Below are a number of issues that often concern young men and women. You will find that some of them are problems or difficulties you have, some are things that are about you but don't concern you, and some may have nothing to do with you.

Read each question in this Inventory carefully. If it expresses something that is a problem for you, MAKE A MARK in the corresponding space next to the number. If the question does not express a difficulty of yours or have to do with you, because it does not happen to you, DO NOT MAKE A MARK; LEAVE IT BLANK.

When you flag an issue, they are saying, "THIS IS A PROBLEM FOR ME, THIS HAPPENS TO ME".

REMINDER:

When you flag an issue they are saying: THIS IS A PROBLEM FOR ME, THIS HAPPENS TO ME".

When you do not mark an issue, and leave it blank, you are saying: "THIS IS NOT A PROBLEM FOR ME, THIS DOES NOT HAPPEN TO ME".

MY PHYSICAL CONDITION OR HEALTH

------ 1-I have a handicapping defect

------ 2-I am concerned about how to improve my figure.

-------3-I am concerned about my health.

------- 4-I get tired easily.

------- 5-I don't get enough sleep.

------ 6-I feel low on energy and energy.

------ 7-Sometimes I feel like I'm going to faint.

------- 8-I would like to know if my energy and stamina are normal.

------- 9-Sometimes I get dizzy.

------- 10-I am always sleepy.

--------11-Sometimes I wet the bed

MY RELATIONSHIPS WITH OTHER BOYS AND GIRLS

------1-I need more friends.

----- 2-I don't make friends with many boys my age.

------3-I don't like other people.

------4- People didn't like it very much

------5-The other guys laugh at me.

------6-I would prefer to play with boys smaller than me.

.00007-I rarely get invitations to go out with friends.

.-----8- I would like to know if my sexual development is normal.

.-----9-Most other boys and girls are selfish to me.

----- 10-The other guys tease me about my size.

.-----11-The other guys tease me because I'm not nice.

.-----12-The other guys tease me about how I look.

-----13-The other guys pick on me because I suck at sports.

----- 14-The other guys tease me because I'm not good at making out.

----- 15-I am afraid to talk to older boys.

-----16-The others treat me like a child.

-----17-I wish I had at least one good friend. MY RELATIONSHIPS WITH

THE SCHOOL.

------1- It is difficult to concentrate

------2- I do not like my current studies.

------3- I hate school.

------4- I would like to quit my studies.

------5-I don't know what I'm studying for.

------6- I don't have good grades.

00007- I forget to do the class work assigned to me.

------8- I am not very smart.

------9- I am too restless and fidgety to stay in class that long.

-----10- It is difficult for me to keep my attention to the class.

-----11-I need help with my studies.

-----12- My teachers make fun of me.

-----13- My teachers are not interested in me.

-----14- My teachers remain very cold and distant.

-----15-My teachers have favorite students.

-----16-My teachers don't understand me

-----17-My teachers don't like me.

-----18- My teachers have it in for me.

-----19- I like this school. ABOUT MYSELF

-----1- I get upset easily.

-----2- I worry about little things.

-----3- I am nervous.

-----4-I can't sleep at night.

-----5-I get distracted a lot because I'm always thinking about nice things that don't exist.

-----6- Sometimes I have thought that life is not worth living.

00007- I feel guilty about things I have done.

-----8- I am not popular among my friends.

-----9- I often feel lonely.

----10- I feel sad and down many times.

----11- I am touchy and easily offended.

----12- I often do things that I later regret.

----13- People notice me a lot.

----14- I guess I'm not as smart as other people.

----15- I prefer to be alone.

----16- I would like to discuss my personal problems with someone.

----17- I would like to know if my mind is functioning normally.

----18- I feel that I am not wanted.

----19- I am concerned about the ugliness or defect of some part of my body.

----20- I have no self-confidence or self-assurance.

----21- I think I'm different from the other guys.

----22- I bite my nails.

----23- Everything goes wrong for me.

----24- I don't know why people get upset or angry with me.

----25- I am afraid of being wrong.

----26- I can't do anything right.

----27- I am fearful.

----28- I almost always need help with the things I do.

----29- I can't stand being told what to do.

----30- I almost always like to do the opposite of what I am told.
----31- I can't stand having to do some things even if they are for the good of my
health.

----32- I tell a lot of lies.

MY HOME AND FAMILY.

----1- I don't get along with my brothers and sisters.

----2- There are constant arguments and fights in my house.

----3- I think I am a burden to my parents.

----4- I cannot discuss my personal affairs with my parents.

----5- I wish Dad was home more.

----6- I wish mom was home more.

00007- I would like to have a brother or sister

----8- My father is domineering and authoritarian.

----9- I feel like I am not part of my family.

----10- I don't like to invite friends to my house-.

----11- My parents have favorites and favorites among their children.

----12- My parents pressure me to study tomorrow what they want and not what I want.

----13- My parents won't let me make my own decisions.

----14- My parents don't trust me

----15- My parents expect too much from me.

----16- I wish my parents wouldn't treat me like a little kid.

----17- I am ashamed of my parents' customs.

----18- I feel like leaving home.

----19- I am afraid to tell my parents that I have committed an offense.

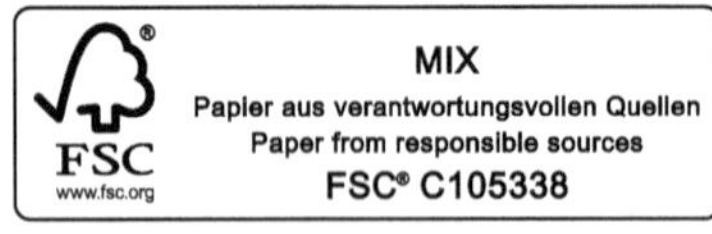

Printed by Books on Demand GmbH, Norderstedt / Germany